ANTIDEPRESSANTS

SOME DOCTORS ARGUE YOUR DOUBTS, THEN THOSE DOCTORS DESTROY YOUR LIFE!!!

BARTHOLOMEW IDENTITY

BALBOA.
PRESS

A DIVISION OF HAY HOUSE

Balboa Press books may be ordered through booksellers or by contacting:

Balboa Press
A Division of Hay House
1663 Liberty Drive
Bloomington, IN 47403
www.balboapress.com.au
1-(877) 407-4847

ISBN: 978-1-4525-0925-9 (sc)
ISBN: 978-1-4525-0926-6 (e)

Because of the dynamic nature of the Internet, any web addresses or links contained in this book may have changed since publication and may no longer be valid. The views expressed in this work are solely those of the author and do not necessarily reflect the views of the publisher, and the publisher hereby disclaims any responsibility for them.

The author of this book does not dispense medical advice or prescribe the use of any technique as a form of treatment for physical, emotional, or medical problems without the advice of a physician, either directly or indirectly. The intent of the author is only to offer information of a general nature to help you in your quest for emotional and spiritual well-being. In the event you use any of the information in this book for yourself, which is your constitutional right, the author and the publisher assume no responsibility for your actions.

Any people depicted in stock imagery provided by Thinkstock are models, and such images are being used for illustrative purposes only.

Certain stock imagery © Thinkstock.

Printed in the United States of America

Balboa Press rev. date: 03/08/2013

CONTENTS

MY ANGRY INTRODUCTION
{MILD-MANNERED}

Because my furious words in this little book will make many professional people very, very angry, there will probably/possibly be a deliberate and violent reaction against my words: to stop YOU from totally finding out what I'm talking about. They will want to go further. They may even try to find out who I am. Therefore I am writing this to you using a pretend identity—which I have named "Bartholomew Identity".

These days, if ANY person says (or prints) ANYTHING which seems to blame someone else for something wrong that has happened (or is happening), then he or she needs to ALWAYS prove that accusation. Everything that I am writing about in this booklet has **already happened** to me! NONE of it is fiction, or pretend (like my identity is pretend). Also I am NEVER going to mention the name of even one living person who has made it hard for me, as I write about this horrible subject.

Regularly (and I actually KNOW that this happens, after talking with the specialist that I used to trust), many of our trusty professional doctors routinely go to "get-togethers". Those "Specialists" pick out different expensive locations on earth to attend their "get-together" conferences. But are you now wondering (like me) what they say about **US** at those meetings?

What I will be going on to describe in this booklet used to be happening to me utterly every day. But I have always realised that I am NOT the only victim of this sort of abuse.

The locking of people away inside thought-prisons—using the excuse the side affects of antidepressants—possibly began in 1961; when the word "antidepressant" was coined!!

Very recently, on Wednesday, 19/12/12, I went to my trusted "specialist". I was quite angry because using Google I had found out that an Antidepressant which I had asked him to prescribe for me contained a dangerous ingredient.

(Please read about shellac on **The Menu as YOU EAT & Supporting References Sheets**—on Pages 14 to 18.)

He had been my trusted psychiatrist for around 12 years. Over that period he had prescribed many, many different antidepressants because after each prescription my appeal was ALWAYS—something was still NOT right.

At my last consultation with him, which I obediently went to (on Wednesday, 19/09/12), I complained that the expensive Antidepressant named "Valdoxan" which I had asked him to let me try out, was not worth the money it cost me to buy! You see for one thing, it was not yet included in the Australian Pharmaceutical Benefit list; and thus I had been required to pay the total damage—**BUT**—even Valdoxan was beginning to prove to be a bit of a dud.

Initially I had noticed that Valdoxan did not make me feel as severely awkward as the earlier antidepressants had done. Also at that time, even though Valdoxan was NOT included in the Australian Pharmaceutical Benefit list, I had decided to go out on a limb—and pay its full price. Not everybody can manage such a pricey commitment but because I could then—I did.

Its cheaper version cost me $62.95 per month for 28 tablets containing 25mg of "Valdoxan".

Then suddenly one day I found out that Valdoxan contains a component named "shellac" that is poisonous to humans!

(Please again read about shellac on **The Menu as YOU EAT & Supporting References Sheets**—on Pages 14 to 18.)

It was because "shellac" sounded like a **<u>very UGLY</u>** "medication" to deliberately be swallowing in order to get better from an illness, that became the "why" that I went tentatively, horrifiedly—and shaking—into Google; the free, common peoples' extant Alexandria Library—to discover the truth about that "medicinal".

Hey, we ALL realise by now that all of the huge Drug Companies need to cover their payroll commitment toward highly-paid staff and high-priced equipment and research—that's business!! For each of the drugs that are designed and manufactured therefore, there is ALWAYS A NEED for a speedy catch-up-with asking price for ALL of their drugs!! Those Drug Companies need to have a guarantee that monies will be on hand for their next medication-invention. BUT do our Western "Doctors" really require (for their professional activity) such a turnover of Antidepressant prescriptions when the inclusion of "shellac" is surely **KNOWN** by doctors to be a dangerous component within any prescription? Should our Western "Doctors" be permitted to so eagerly go along with the contents of a medication, even when they MUST professionally utterly recognise an endangerment to human health?

Difficult for me to believe (and hard for me to bear) recently was the reaction of my then psychiatrist when I mentioned my anxiety about the shellac. You see, his only reaction was that his eyes became incredibly lifeless—and then he changed the subject!!!

But this exposure will **NOT** become lifeless—and he will **NOT** change the subject in here!!!

No!!!!

I'm mad about this! Compare me to a frenzied, speared bull in an arena—just before the sword (the "estoque") is driven between its shoulders to kill it. Never will I allow this bone of contention of mine to be ditched by one of those professionals during a consultation—**EVER** again!

I will cover that wager by **NEVER** again allowing a Western psychiatrist Doctor to, like a fattened blowfly, even "**see**" me, so that those blowflies of that category will NOT be able to lay their maggots on me—**EVER** again!!

MY INCENSED PREFACE
{INSULTABLY INDIGNANT}

To avoid an early and painful, potent termination of my enraged procedure to remove the manhole cover of this disgraceful sewer which penetrates and permeates human societies, human families, members that are our precious, precocious infants—to our treasured, dignity-seeking elderly—I am writing this under the nom de plume: "Bartholomew Identity".

Also, to avoid avertable legitimate legal repercussions, unless I am quoting from another source (which will be **always perceptible** by my use of distinct references and the appropriate punctuation), <u>**NEVER**</u> will I mention even **one sole human person's name** in relation to the burden I have endured and sought succour for via Western Medical Practitioners since 1964; and needed (actually) since I was very young.

At the regular "Sanctioned-Doctors Only" Conventions held at diverse, global, extravagant venues; do those wealthy members beam out there each time with the excited catchphrase mantra: "The only thing that stops a tired guy with a "depressed" (actually this simply means dispirited, downcast) appearance is a medical guy with a prescription for antidepressants!!??"

The scenario, which I am in this booklet depicting, was once my prevailing, appalling reality; however I know that I am **NOT** a sole victim; thus my hideous internment had **NOT** been unique!

This type of incarceration by the effect of Antidepressants (which is often almost laughingly, nearly callously, verbally mitigated by the delivery of the terminology, "side-affects") has been a legally enacted operant of Medical professionals at least since the first known use of even the word "antidepressant"—in 1961.

Only a few months ago, Wednesday, 19/09/12, I fronted up to a consultation with a doctor. Because I had bizarrely (my personal, innate reflexing) discovered an ingredient in the Valdoxan antidepressant (which I'd already been faithfully swallowing for many months)—and which I did **<u>NOT</u>** need to be a brain specialist (nor a GP) to dread the wallop of upon my already polluted body's system—is poisonous!! My survival mechanisms; which by nature are within each one of us—had become extraordinarily regenerated—this time with the effectualness of my very fierce emotionalism.

Over the twelve years of being "seen" by my (then current) psychiatrist—many, many drugging antidepressant prescriptions had been issued out to me; because of today's multi-numerous lashings of alternative antidepressant highways.

Most recently I had been professionally allowed the liberty to actually quit administering myself with that antidepressant named "Valdoxan". The cost factor thereat which personally affected me (a then "depressed" pensioner) was significant, because at the time Valdoxan was **NOT** included on the Australian Pharmaceutical Benefit list!

Yet, because Valdoxan was an remarkably less-posture-crippling alternative, and because I am/was in the fortunate financial position to carry that (contaminated) load solely upon my shoulders (in its generic version); I thus for more than six months resolutely and quite keenly paid the necessary $62.95 per month for 28 of the 25mg tablets called Valdoxan.

One day, right out of the blue, I discovered that "Valdoxan" contains an ingredient named "shellac".

Because that sounded quite toxic to me I went onto the net and, yes, it **IS** a questionable product for a human to be deliberately swallowing; particularly when still under the caring, medical guidance—of a "doctor".

Here's what I found out via Google!

(Please again read that on **The Menu as YOU EAT & Supporting References Sheets**—Pages 14 to 18.)

However apart from that obvious and typical amoral (of course, in my prescription-case-particular) Drug Company's fast-buck act of the nonchalant, impersonal production of such a "medicine"—should also the quick consultation turnover of human patients be so vital to our Western doctors that a substance known as shellac has been medically-acceptably incorporated within some of their patient's prescriptions—and should they so eagerly actually obviously concur that such a drug formulation be morally and ethically prescribable?

Incredibly, the mention however, of that shellac-concern of mine to "my psychiatrist" was met by the nonchalant opacity of his gaze; and the matter was abruptly dumped by his professionally changing of the subject.

Not dumped any longer!!

No!!!

Driven and resolved to continue to be driven, I will **NOT** allow this subject to be dumped again; because I will **NOT EVER** consult with him; nor will I consult with any others of his professional fraternity again; and via the assistance from a reputable Publisher, am making this chronic horror-story of mine very, very public.

CHAPTER 1A

THE CURTAIN RISES LIKE THIS
{MILD MANNERED}

It was purely by chance that I had spotted the shellac.

After getting wind of that 'legal fiction'-like attack against my health and well-being, I began to wonder about the possibility of other harmful components being prescribed to go down through my gullet and into my stomach.

At the end of that "shellac" consultation, that Western Specialist doctor prescribed an alternative antidepressant named Deptram.

Doxepin tablets, 50 mg.

(Please read A Bit About "Deptram" {Reference A}, and A Bit About "Deptram" {Reference B} on **The Menu as YOU EAT & Supporting References Sheets**—on Pages 12 to 14.)

Thanks to information on the Internet—taken from some main sites like [>>http://en.wikipedia.org/wiki/Main_Page<<] and the dictionary source site [>>http://www.onelook.com/<<] and many, **many** other wonderful, revealing, free Internet sites—now I can know the exact meaning of every word that the specialists and the GPs bounce around about so-called

"Depression"—and so would and will **YOU**—and every other human—**NOW** be enabled to know!! Keep looking!!!

It could never be, that the Lecturers in each of humanity's vital universities—who are morally and ethically devoted to explain the perils that are always holding the line, if a doctor prescribes a wrong medication—would neglect to encourage the practice of a **MoralEthic Code**.

For how long, in your case, have you been enduring **YOUR** personal horror-story. The "Legal Practitioner" who wrote out the prescription that YOU should now regimentally swallow to get better—does he or she just have deaf ears when you say how difficult the side-effects of the "medication" are to cope with? Does he or she perhaps also even have a bit of a chuckle (even while you are still actually sitting in front of him or her, in his or her consulting room) about the fact that you are putting on weight; or that you are always feeling dizzy, and your face is numb; or that you are not able to get a good night's sleep; or that your voice is always slurred when you talk to **ANYONE—ALL THE TIME**; or that you are always constipated?

In my case, my feeling of wonder and admiration for the modern humans who had studied hard at a university was huge! I used to think these must be extremely-committed humans who then had altruistically decided to become Medical Practitioners—and so now they were obviously also rightly legally authorised to prescribe the latest chemicals combined within a capsule or a pill or a lozenge that are so wonderfully developed and produced by modern, superstar Chemists who work for our very marvellous, ultramodern, selfless Pharmaceutical Companies!

But it was very soon after I had put all of my trust in **all** of those empires (setup for the medical salvation of humanity) that I began to feel the shock of a very clumsy betrayal of my trust, by those wonderful innovative peoples!! I fairly quickly turned into a fumbling, gawky, stumbling and dribbling and traumatised man; and therefore soon became both unemployable—and a socially even **more-useless** member of the Australian population.

If any observer tossed this bizarre jumble of cruel human problems over in their mind (like tossing a salad of different vegetables) they would definitely be able to quickly/easily recognise the vicious cycle of the miss-tossing of a few of the members of the salad—that are **all members of our human Family**. And if then that watching person decided to look into this mess more closely, he or she would be appalled to realise also that what they had just perceived was only the tip of a typically-mostly-invisible, grievous titanic iceberg!!

From vague memory (vague because I'm nearly 65 now), when I was only 10 I was already struggling with life, because it was as though I was expected to be pushing a heavily-loaded wheelbarrow that was on a very skinny wheel, up a very steep sandy hillside. Talking about the real world with other people was very difficult; anyway what was reality? Probably because I was obviously a complicated little onion, even my Dad had little time for me. My Mum and I were very close (when we got the chance to be); but because she and Dad had built a shop, even she was hard to pin down, and to talk to; because that business had been a 7 days per week (and very busy) operation.

Can you recall that when you were a kid (like I can) you enjoyed the bubbling, vigorous anticipation of wanting to also fly like the gorgeous little willy-wagtails and the budgerigars? But now, like I can, can you also remember those weird times when you found it hard to even keep up with your mates? I used to helplessly wonder then—what is wrong with me?

Can **YOU** also remember times like that?

CHAPTER 1B

ALSO, THE CURTAIN RISES LIKE THIS
{INSULTABLY INDIGNANT}

It had been only by happenstance that I had spotted the shellac.

And, thereafter to now, during reflection upon that pervasion . . . what else that I had been believing-in and thence countenancing by swallowing, had been likewise ambushing me with similar sinister ancillaries??

Meanwhile, at that appointment on Wednesday, 19/09/12, with almost over-confident alacrity, that Specialist adverted and, yes, actually **re**-prescribed Deptran (Doxepin tablets, 50 mg)—an antidepressant that **HE KNEW** had caused me woes in the past.

Because of the debilitated state I was still then being crushed by on 19/09/12, **I** could not (at that time) recall my initial (I do recall now, hideous) experience with it.

(Again, please read A Bit About "Deptram" {Reference A}, and A Bit About "Deptram" {Reference B} on **The Menu as YOU EAT & Supporting References Sheets**—on Pages 12 to 14.)

Because of being the fatigued, gullible increasingly-aging fool which I was wont to be after the many decades of my credulous, submissive trust of all neurology-degree-brandishing medical practitioners—and the resultant flushing of my cognisance of all (**possibly within-even-me, and which is normally-existent in all humans**) valuable common sense—and stultified by multi-prescriptions of antidepressants—I was never able then to even envisage the true scenario; let alone, as now, "see (**in sharp focus**) the whole (**very ugly**) picture"!

Thanks to the Internet's care delivery to me of [>>http://en.wikipedia.org/wiki/Main_Page<<] and [>>http://www.onelook.com/<<] and many, **many** other sites, now I can consider the distinct meaning of every dictionary word; and herein this topic, the foisting of a/this trickery by intolerant, impatient professionals upon the current whole civilisation of humans!!

Most-surely, every last "chuckle" of this truly-frightening imbroglio directed toward **ALL** of humanity does **NOT** commence behind the "closed doors" of medical universities? However do the Pharmacology Lecturers in those noble institutions also sufficiently caution that theatre of eager pupils about the necessary very cautious precautions—and the requirement of the application of very moral ethics—when recommending powerful, potentially-further-debilitating medications to other humans via prescriptions?

For how long by now has an increasingly-familiar, yes in fact **universal**, horror-story—**perhaps even this very same story, with YOU in it instead of me**—been crippling your competency and your cosmopolitan rights to sanity; and your universal rights to your physical health?

Deceptively the initial "awe" of whatever was first off recommended in my case, to solve my struggle with life—was a prescribed, benumbing antidepressant "silver bullet"; actually more than just one. But that inaugural wonderment sorserised chop chop into the desperate shock of its seriously-embarrassing playfellow—severely benumbed, inelegant consummate dribbling cack-handedness.

And as anyone might have despondently reflected upon our (we "depressed" persons) banishment from normal life by those briefly depicted symptoms; also we guinea pigs might too have perceived that, monstrously, those resultant indicants are just the tip of a towering, hidden-below-the-waves, titanic and seemingly-fated apparently (presently!!) inescapable misfortune.

Even from as early as when I was a 10 year-old boy, for a then unknown "why?", I torpidly adjudicated within my quorum of only one—that it was far too difficult to relate with most other humans; even my Dad. On the contrary my Mum and I were always very connected, but she was always, with Dad, constantly detoured from me (actually from all of us 3 kids) by the requirement to take care of their large shop.

Within my enervated world then, I could not have foreseen this time period now; nor the gold of being able to bring into focus, and comprehend that Einstein's equation deducting the energy that is acquirable from matter—and herein pertaining to a human's resource of healthy, abundant sentience—also depends upon the degree of tappable radiance of it when it is appertaining to a human person's resultant mental and physical energy.

Without doubt surely, it could be totally criminally **WRONG** for some university graduates to set up a "Practise" and thereafter begin to legally potentially devastate the lives of other vulnerable, trusting humans!!

Often (even while we common people are noticing an obvious attempt to steer our attention away from it), we are actually seeing and hearing some influential, important person put his/her foot in it by saying—or doing—something blatantly, very obviously totally inappropriate.

When a sick person with serious coping problems goes for help to a doctor, **even we common people recognise** that it is very, very wrong for that legally registered "doctor" to knowingly prescribe a medication which (they **MUST** however at the very least **suspect**) just might make a serious problem related with coping with our personal problems in life even **WORSE**!!!!

There are a great many humans on the same earth WE all call home who are starving to death because they have NO food. We common people naturally react in helpless horror!! But what sort of reaction would we common people feel and unavoidably noisily display because of their starvation (and such an intervention)—if Western doctors were given even **MORE** power over human destinies; and some of those Western doctors went surging forward (even more out of **MoralEthic** control than they are now), and implemented a procedure ensuring that all of the starving ones were speedily, more conveniently, prescribed antidepressants—instead of being **immediately** given food and water and safe shelter?!!

Within the Mirriam Webster Internet site [>>http://www.merriam-webster.com/<<] there is a definition of the word "antidepressant" at [>>http://www.merriam-webster.com/dictionary/antidepressant<<].

There we can read that an antidepressant is: (Please read that on **The Menu as YOU EAT & Supporting References Sheets**—on Pages 19 & 20.)

- Continued on page 21 -

THE FOREWORD [>>http://www.bpsbooks.com/BPS-Books-blog/bid/21727/What-s-the-Difference-Between-a-Foreword-Preface-and-Introduction<<]

"A foreword (one of the most often misspelled words in the language) is most often written by someone other than the author: an expert in the field, a writer of a similar book, etc. Forewords help the publisher at the level of marketing: An opening statement by an eminent and well-published author gives them added credibility in pitching the book to bookstores. Forewords help the author by putting a stamp of approval on their work."

Well, this is the author of "**Antidepressants—Some Doctors Argue Your Doubts, Then Those Doctors Destroy Your Life**", Bartholomew Identity speaking (writing).

Unfortunately, possibly even for me, obviously I am **NOT** eminent.

Also, possibly unfortunately, I am not only **not** well-published—in fact I am NOT published **AT ALL**—in truth, I used to be categorised as "Majorly-Depressed" and sometimes "Bi-polarly-Depressed"!!!

However, I hereby dare to interpenetrate the qualifications of the Foreword-statement-penners as I fabricate **MY OWN** darn ardent foreword; as follows:

MY FOREWORD

Some people might belong to "The Ministry of Silly Walks"; as is evoked in "a sketch from the Monty Python comedy troupe's television show **Monty Python's Flying Circus**, episode 14". [>>http://en.wikipedia.org/wiki/The_Ministry_of_Silly_Walks<<]

The "Ministry" I believe that **I** might belong to may be called, say, "Ministry of Unwieldy Talks".

We are **MANY**!!!!!!

We of that impressive "Ministry" eagerly and zealously do accept the superlative responsibility of most respectfully harkening **ALL** (in utter toto) to the delectable, proud 17th Century English syntax utilisation of our pride-instilling, awesomely-majestic lexicon.

The Menu as YOU Eat & Supporting References Sheets—*Sheet 2 of 12*

That appreciative heeding of our Ministry MUST be not only savoured—for a full appreciation of it, it **MUST** be individually delivered!

Compriato?!!

Getting to the point; as I am **many** times, and **sometimes** even professionally, gently **urged** to do (I should wonder "why?!!!"):

In this Middle-of-the-Work Foreword of **MINE** (by yours truly, Bartholomew Identity), I must now let you know that the **utter urgency** of what is contained inside here must **NEVER** be attenuated by, perhaps, another one's dislike of (or snigger towards) 17th Century-type tok (Respected American enunciation of the English word "talk")!! [>>http://www.thefreedictionary.com/enunciate<<]

A passing thought: How wonderfully—and delightfully—dissimilar are we all!

Inside here (this "**Antidepressants—Some Doctors Argue Your Doubts, Then Those Doctors Destroy Your Life**" booklet), I **DO** repeat themes.

Please **DO NOT** be annoyed by this.

A very young person who might notice this booklet on sale somewhere—and feels motivated because of its accusative title to pick it up and peer into it—needs to then be hastened to take a deeper plunge—and grab this booklet to the extent of ownership; and take it home and delve into it more profoundly.

However what very young person has sufficiently developed a "Ministry" love for my inferior interlingual rendition of 17th Century enunciation??

Consequently with that pivotal factor in my mind, I have **first-presented** paragraphs in "Today"-talk (incorporating my best, **non-eminent** ability); and/but then I have also gone and **repeated** those paragraphs using the 17th Century mainlining language (to my best, **non-eminent** ability) for my superior compatriots.

We are all striving for a place, somewhere!

Also, because you have **not** been acquainted prior to this focus, my Booklet-partitions are:

[A] **MY FOREWORD** (written above, on page 9.),

[B] **MY ANGRY INTRODUCTION** (the first section within the covers; written on pages vii to ix.),

[C] **MY INCENSED PREFACE** (a 17th Century paraphrasing of that same "first" section; written on pages xi to xiii.),

[D] **CHAPTER 1A—THE CURTAIN RISES LIKE THIS** (the first existent chapter within the covers; written on pages 1 to 3.),

[E] **CHAPTER 1B—ALSO, THE CURTAIN RISES LIKE THIS** (a 17th Century paraphrasing of that same "first" existent chapter; written on pages 5 to 8.),

[F] **The Menu as YOU EAT & Critical References Pages** (14 essential, one-stop reference sheets; written on pages 9 to 22.),

[G] **CHAPTER 2A—THE CURTAIN FALLS** (the second existent chapter within the covers; written on pages 23 & 24.),

[H] **CHAPTER 2B—THE CURTAIN FALLS WITH A LOUD THUMP** (a 17th Century paraphrasing of that same "second" existent chapter; written on page 25.),

[I] **MY SOLUTION** (The medicine that alleviates my Fatigue; written on page 27.),

[J] **MY CONCLUSION** (A summary of breathtakingly comparative principles; written on pages 29 & 30—and which includes two Tables.)

The **MOST OUTSTANDING** purpose of my "**not** eminent" (I'm just an aged "commoner" pensioner, whom has now actually whiteouted his "disability"!) endeavour is to shout out loudly to every human on this earth who can read—whether preferring to read simple peeved straight talk, or insultably the 17th Century, more elevated, syntax—by squalling this: We humans are (in reality) no more important to many Western doctors than the ruthlessly expendable Cavia cobayas—those tailless guinea pigs that are "used" during medical research!!!!

A Bit About "Deptram" {Reference A}

"Deptran is used to treat depression. Deptran 10 mg and Deptran 25 mg capsules can be used at any stage in the treatment of depression. However, the higher strength, Deptran 50 mg tablets, is approved only for the maintenance treatment of depression (after your symptoms have improved)." [>>http://www.itsmyhealth.com.au/medicines/deptran<<]

A Bit About "Deptram" {Reference B}

"Doxepin was first synthesized in the 1960s. If doxepin is used chronically during pregnancy, the newborn may show a withdrawal syndrome with agitation, impaired cardio-respiratory functions, disturbed urination and defecation. Caution should be exerted in treating pregnant women on a regular basis. Doxepin is found in significant amounts in the milk of lactating women. If therapy is necessary, breastfeeding should be interrupted during treatment. In order to maintain supply, the mother may pump and discard the milk during her treatment.

"**Central Nervous System**: fatigue, dizziness, drowsiness, lightheadedness, confusion, nightmares, agitation, increased anxiety, insomnia, seizures (infrequently), delirium, rarely induction of hypomania and schizophrenia (stop medication immediately), extrapyramidal side-effects (rarely), abuse in patients with polytoxikomania (rarely), tinnitus;

"**Anticholinergic**: dry mouth, constipation, even ileus (rarely), difficulties in urinating, sweating, precipitation (acceleration) of glaucoma;

"**Antiadrenergic**: hypotension, postural collapse (if patient arises too fast from lying/sitting position to standing), arrhythmias (sinus-tachycardia, bradycardia, av-blockade);

"**Allergic/toxic**: skin rash, photosensitivity, liver damage of the cholostatic type (rarely), hepatitis (extremely rare), leuko—or thrombopenia (rarely), agranulocytosis (very rarely), hypoplastic anemia (rarely);

"**Others**: frequently increased appetite, weight gain, rarely nausea, frequently impaired sexual function in men (impotence, ejaculation-difficulties), rarely hypertension, rarely polyneuropathy, in both sexes breast-enlargement and galactorrhea (rarely). May increase or decrease liver function in some patients.

"Other remarks:

Doxepin may worsen psychotic conditions like schizophrenia and should be given with caution; the antipsychotic treatment should be continued.

"**With Zonalon and Xepin**: in most countries an external form (cream) is available for the treatment of itching skin disease; the effect is probably due to the affinity of doxepin for H1 and H2 receptors and action on muscarinic receptors. Doxepin is the most anxiolytic of all the tricyclic antidepressants.

"Pharmacology:

Doxepin inhibits the reuptake of serotonin and norepinephrine. Its actions of the reuptake of dopamine are negligible. Doxepin also has antagonistic effects at a variety of receptors." [>>http://en.wikipedia.org/wiki/Doxepin<<]

Ouch, ouch, ouch; but were NOT done yet!!!

"DEPTRAN SIDE EFFECTS

Deptran is a dibenzoxepin tricyclic compound that is prescribed for the treatment of depression. It is called tricyclic because its chemical structure contains three rings. Deptran's mechanism of action is unknown. Deptran is available as a capsule and also as a mint-flavoured oral concentrate in liquid.

"Systemic Side Effects

According to a 2004 study by Kenneth Wilson and Pat Mottram published in the "International Journal of Geriatric Psychiatry," gastrointestinal side effects are experienced at a higher rate in those taking classical tricyclic antidepressants, compared to those taking selective serotonin reuptake inhibitors. They are also associated with significantly higher withdrawal rates. Some of these side effects include constipation and nausea. Other side effects may involve difficulty or frequent urination, dry mouth and excessive sweating.

"Neurological Effects

There are some neurological side effects associated with this medication. These may include drowsiness, weakness, tiredness, nightmares or blurred vision. The drowsiness tends to decrease and disappear over the course of treatment. While taking this medicine, skin may be more sensitive to sunlight. Changes in sex drive or ability or changes in appetite or weight are other potential side effects.

"Muscle or Gait Problems

More serious side effects of Deptran use include muscle or gait problems. Muscle problems may include back, neck and jaw muscle spasms. Gait issues related to Deptran use are characterized by a shuffling walk or uncontrollable shaking in a body part. The heart may also be affected, in the form of an irregular heartbeat. These symptoms should be reported to a physician." [>>http://www.livestrong.com/article/256342-deptran-side-effects/<<]

TOXICITY OF SHELLAC

"SHELLAC POISONING

This is poisoning from swallowing shellac. This is for information only and not for use in the treatment or management of an actual poison exposure. If you have an exposure, you should call your local emergency number (such as 911) or the National Poison Control Center at 1-800-222-1222.

"Poisonous Ingredient

> Ethanol
> Isopropanol

> Methanol
> Methyl isobutyl ketone

"Where Found

> Paint remover
> Shellac
> Wood finishing products

"**Note:** This '**Where Found**' list may not be all-inclusive.

"Symptoms

Eyes, ears, nose, and throat

> Blindness
> Blurred vision
> Wide pupils

"Heart and blood

> Convulsions
> Disturbance of the acid balance of the blood (leads to multi-organ failure)
> Low blood pressure

"Kidneys

> Kidney failure

"Lungs and airways

> No breathing
> Rapid, shallow breathing

The Menu as YOU Eat & Supporting References Sheets—*Sheet 8 of 12*

"Muscles

> Leg cramps
> Weakness

"Nervous system

> Coma
> Dizziness
> Fatigue
> Headache

"Skin

> Cyanosis (blue skin, lips, or fingernails)

"Stomach and intestines

> Diarrhoea
> Nausea
> Vomiting

"Home Care

Do NOT make a person throw up unless told to do so by poison control or a health care professional. Seek immediate medical help.

If the chemical is on the skin or in the eyes, flush with lots of water for at least 15 minutes.

If the chemical was swallowed, immediately give the person water, unless instructed otherwise by a health care provider. Do NOT give water if the patient is having symptoms (such as vomiting, convulsions, or a decreased level of alertness) that make it hard to swallow.

"Before Calling Emergency

Determine the following information:

> Patient's age, weight, and condition
> Name of the product (ingredients and strengths, if known)
> Time it was swallowed
> Amount swallowed

"Poison Control

The National Poison Control Center (1-800-222-1222) can be called from anywhere in the United States. This national hotline number will let you talk to experts in poisoning. They will give you further instructions.

This is a free and confidential service. All local poison control centers in the United States use this national number. You should call if you have any questions about poisoning or poison prevention. It does NOT need to be an emergency. You can call for any reason, 24 hours a day, 7 days a week.

Take the container with you to the hospital, if possible.

See: **Poison control center—emergency number**

"What to Expect at the Emergency Room

The health care provider will measure and monitor the patient's vital signs, including temperature, pulse, breathing rate, and blood pressure. Symptoms will be treated as appropriate. The patient may receive:

> Breathing tube
> Bronchoscopy—camera down the throat to see burns in the airways and lungs
> Endoscopy—camera down the throat to see burns in the esophagus and the stomach
> Hemodialysis

The Menu as YOU Eat & Supporting References Sheets—*Sheet 10 of 12*

> Fluids through a vein (IV)
> Medicine (antidote) to reverse the effect of the poison
> Oxygen
> Surgical removal of burned skin (skin debridement)
> Tube through the mouth into the stomach to wash out the stomach (gastric lavage)
> Washing of the skin (irrigation)—perhaps every few hours for several days

"Outlook (Prognosis)

Isopropanol and methanol are extremely poisonous. As little as 2 tablespoons of methanol can kill a child, while 2 to 8 ounces can be deadly for adults.

How well a patient does depends on the amount of poison swallowed and how quickly treatment was received. The faster a patient gets medical help, the better the chance for recovery.

"References

Jacobsen D, Hovda KE. Methanol, ethylene glycol, and other toxic alcohols. In: Shannon MW, Borron SW, Burns MJ, eds. Haddad and Winchester's Clinical Management of Poisoning and Drug Overdose. 4th ed. Philadelphia, Pa: Saunders Elsevier; 2007:chap 32.

"Update Date: 2/28/2012

Updated by: Eric Perez, MD, St. Luke's / Roosevelt Hospital Center, NY, NY, and Pegasus Emergency Group (Meadowlands and Hunterdon Medical Centers), NJ. Review provided by VeriMed Healthcare

Network. Also reviewed by David Zieve, MD, MHA, Medical Director, A.D.A.M., Inc."

[>>http://www.nlm.nih.gov/medlineplus/ency/article/002821.htm<<]

On ABC2, Tuesday morning 21/01/13 after 12:30 AM AEST, a documentary was re-aired; and this time entitled "The True Story".

"'All Watched Over by Machines of Loving Grace' is a 2011 BBC documentary series by filmmaker Adam Curtis. The series argues that computers have failed to liberate humanity and instead have "distorted and simplified our view of the world around us". The title is taken from the 1967 poem of the same name by Richard Brautigan. The first of three episodes aired on Monday 23 May 2011 at 9pm on BBC2.

"In the first episode {'Love and Power'}, Curtis tracks the effects of Ayn Rand's ideas on American financial markets, particularly via the influence on Alan Greenspan.

"This episode {the second episode of Curtis' three episodes} investigates how machine ideas such as cybernetics and systems theory were applied to natural ecosystems, and how this relates to the false idea that there is a balance of nature. Cybernetics has been applied to human beings to attempt to build societies without central control, self organising networks built of people, based on a fantasy view of nature.

"This programme {the third episode of Curtis' three episodes—'The Monkey In The Machine and the Machine in the Monkey'} looked into the selfish gene theory which holds that humans are machines controlled by genes which was invented by William Hamilton. Adam Curtis also covered the source of ethnic conflict that was created by Belgian colonialism's artificial creation of a racial divide and the ensuing slaughter that occurred in the Democratic Republic of the Congo, which is a source of raw material for computers and cell phones.

"Interviews and reviews

In May 2011, Adam Curtis was interviewed about the series by Katharine Viner in The Guardian, by the Register and by Little Atoms.

Catherine Gee at the Daily Telegraph said that what Adam Curtis "reveals is the dangers of human beings at their most selfish and self-satisfying. Showing no compassion or consideration for your fellow human beings creates a chasm between those able to walk over others and those too considerate—or too short-sighted—to do so."

The Menu as YOU Eat & Supporting References Sheets—*Sheet 12 of 12*

John Preston also reviewed the first episode, and said that although it showed flashes of brilliance it had an "infuriating glibness too as the web of connectedness became ever more stretched. No one could dispute that Curtis has got a very big bite indeed. But what about the chewing, you ask. There wasn't any—or nothing like enough of it to prevent a bad case of mental indigestion."

Andrew Anthony published a review in The Observer and The Guardian, and commented on the central premise that we had been made to "believe we could create a stable world that would last for ever" but that he doesn't "recall ever believing that "we" could create a stable world that would last for ever", and noted that: "For the film-maker there seems to be an objective reality that a determined individual can penetrate if he is willing to challenge the confining chimeras of markets and machines. Forget the internet tycoons. The Randian hero is Curtis himself."" [Part quotation of: >>http://en.wikipedia.org/wiki/All_Watched_Over_by_Machines_of_Loving_Grace_%28TV_series%29<<]

DEFINITION OF "ANTIDEPRESSANT"

"Any drug used to treat depression. The three main types inhibit the metabolism of serotonin and norepinephrine in the brain. The aim is to keep these monoamine neurotransmitters from dropping to levels associated with depression. The drugs may take a few weeks to show any effect. Tricyclic antidepressants, which inhibit inactivation of norepinephrine and serotonin, help more than 70% of patients. Monoamine oxidase (MAO) inhibitors apparently block the action of MAO, an enzyme that helps break down norepinephrine, serotonin, and dopamine in neurons. They have unpredictable side effects and are usually given only when tricyclic drugs do not help. Selective serotonin reuptake inhibitors (SSRIs) apparently block reabsorption only of serotonin, allowing its levels to build up in the brain. SSRIs, which include fluoxetine (trade name Prozac), often help with depression unrelieved by tricyclics or MAO inhibitors and have milder side effects."

- Continued from page 8 -

Thanks to information on the Internet—taken from some main sites like [>>http://en.wikipedia.org/wiki/Main_Page<<] and the dictionary source site [>>http://www.onelook.com/<<] and many, many other wonderful, revealing, free Internet sites—now I can know the exact meaning of every word that the specialists and the GPs bounce around about so-called "Depression"—and so would and will **YOU**—and every other human—**NOW** be reenabled to know!!

It could never be, that the Lecturers in each of humanity's vital universities—whom are morally and ethically also-devoted to explain the perils that are always holding the line, if a doctor prescribes a wrong medication—would neglect to encourage the practice of a **MoralEthic Code**.

For how long, in your case, have you been enduring YOUR personal horror-story? The "Legal Practitioner" who wrote out the prescription that YOU should now regimentally swallow to get better—does he or she just have deaf ears when you say how difficult the side-effects of the "medication" are to cope with? Does he or she perhaps also even have a bit of a chuckle (even while you are still actually sitting in front of him or her, in his or her consulting room) about the fact that you are putting on weight; or that you are always feeling dizzy, and your face is numb; or that you are not able to get a good night's sleep; or that your voice is always slurred when you talk to **ANYONE—ALL THE TIME**; or that you are always constipated?

In my case, my feeling of wonder and admiration for the modern humans who had studied hard at a university was huge! I used to think these must be extremely-committed humans whom then had altruistically decided to become Medical Practitioners—and so now they were obviously also rightly legally authorised to prescribe the latest chemicals combined within a capsule or a pill or a lozenge that are so wonderfully developed and produced by modern, superstar Chemists who work for our very marvellous, ultramodern, selfless Pharmaceutical Companies!

But it was very soon after I had put all of my trust in all of those empires (which had been setup for the medical salvation of humanity) that I began to feel the shock of a very clumsy betrayal of my trust, by those wonderful innovative peoples!! I fairly quickly turned into a fumbling, gawky, stumbling and dribbling and traumatised man; and therefore, not long after, became both unemployable—and a socially **even more-pathetic** member of the Australian population.

If any observer tossed this bizarre jumble of cruel human problems over in their mind (like tossing a salad of different vegetables) they would definitely be able to quickly/easily recognise the vicious cycle of the miss-tossing of a few of the members of the salad—that (whom) are all members of **our human Family**. And if then that watching person decided to look into this mess more closely, he or she would be appalled to realise also that what they had just perceived was only the tip of a typically-mostly-invisible, devastating titanic iceberg!!

From vague memory (vague because I'm nearly 65 now), when I was only 10 I was already struggling with life, because it was as though I was expected to be pushing a heavily-loaded wheelbarrow that was on a knife-edged wheel, up a very steep, extinctioned sandy hillside. Talking about the real world with other people was very difficult; anyway what was reality? Probably because I was obviously a complicated little onion, even my Dad had little time for me. My Mum and I were very close (when we got the chance to be); but because she and Dad had built a retailing premises, even **she** was hard to pin down, and to talk to; because that business had been a 7 days per week and extremely-engaged micro-emporium.

Can you recall that when you were a kid (like I can) you enjoyed the bubbling, vigorous anticipation of wanting to also wing and hover like the gorgeous little willy-wagtails and the budgerigars? But now, like I can, can you also remember those weirdly, seriously-awkward times when you found it hard to even keep up with your peers? I used to helplessly, puerilely wonder then—what is wrong with me?

Can **YOU** also impotently recollect saddening times like that?

CHAPTER 2A

THE CURTAIN FALLS
{MILD-MANNERED}

If a person appears to be worn-out it could be because he/she is not eating enough good food, or perhaps he/she burns his/her candle at both ends. Some problem is depriving he/she of energy.

Without anyone understanding this subject matter in the 1950s, there was I (just a kid) desperately searching for energy as I tried to find a life.

Without doubt surely, it would be totally criminally **WRONG** for some university graduates to set up a "Practise" and thereafter begin to legally potentially devastate the lives of other vulnerable, trusting humans!!

Often (even while we common people are noticing an obvious attempt to steer our attention away from it), we are actually seeing and hearing some influential, important person put his/her foot in it by saying—or doing—something blatantly, very obviously totally inappropriate.

When a sick person with serious coping problems goes for help to a doctor, even we common people recognise that it is very, very wrong for that legally registered "doctor" to knowingly prescribe a medication which (they may suspect, however) just might make a serious problem related with coping with our personal problems in life even **WORSE**!!!!

There are a great many humans on the same earth WE all call home who are starving to death because they have NO food. We common people naturally react in helpless horror!! But what sort of reaction would we feel and unavoidably display because of their starvation (and such an intervention), if Western doctors were given even **MORE** power over human destinies; and some of those Western doctors went surging forward (even more out of **MoralEthic control** than they are now), and ensured that all of the starving ones were speedily, more conveniently, prescribed antidepressants—instead of being immediately given food and water and safe shelter?!!

Within the Mirriam Webster Internet site [>>http://www.merriam-webster.com/<<] there is a definition of the word "antidepressant" at [>>http://www.merriam-webster.com/dictionary/ antidepressant<<].

(Please read that on **The Menu as YOU EAT & Supporting References Pages**—on Pages 19 & 20.)

CHAPTER 2B

THE CURTAIN FALLS WITH A LOUD THUMP
{INSULTABLY-INDIGNANT}

If there is NOT some glimmer of energy there is, at the very least, the confirmed possibility of a historicism of no derivable mass-energy source!!

That state, one of diminished energy, must have been the dominant factor hindering me, ever since early childhood.

So, very-emphatically, is it not wholly **IMPROPER** to proceed to prescribe (via antidepressants or whatever) a benumbing of any fatigued victim's otherwise very normal (that person being already exasperated and exacerbated by his/her terrifying debilitation) apprehensions about tomorrow (especially these days)—and then also effectively go ahead to possibly drug-induce an emotional false flux of confusing, intermittent complacence within that person!??

We are from time to time cognisant of eye—and ear-witnessing at least the occasional bungled lurch of even our most mentally-healthy, responsibility-assimilated leaders; perchance THEY—no one is perfect—become clumsily complacent in some area during their pursuits.

However to oblige a casualty whom has "presented" with a chronicle of serious difficulties pertaining to his/her **NON**-successes in life, and to his/her **INABILITY** to customise his/her own self-confidence—and **retain** his/her own "self-confidence"—**IS IT NOT A SERIOUS CRIME** by **ANY** prescriber against every one of their patient´s recourse to humanity—to then go and further professionally incapacitate that suffering human; by plying **ANY** class of (by the prescriber, personally and most-definitely shied away from) chemical stupefaction agency??!!!!

Earth´s world's population of those whom are media-familiarised (and empathetic) witnesses to the effects of malnutrition upon **ANY** human child's hopes and **ANY** adult human´s prescience, are continuously and limitlessly, unendingly horrified by scenes of starvation! But then what would be the reaction of we cognisant adult global witnesses, if also **THOSE** circumstantially assailed starving victims were purposely initially administered with antidepressants—instead of being determinatively, solely facilitated toward the repairing of their organic, physical being; and a concerted eager attempt made to provide them with just plain, regular food and ample water and a safe home?!!

At the Mirriam Webster [>>http://www.merriam-webster.com/<<] site; at its [>>http://www.merriam-webster.com/dictionary/antidepressant<<] furnishing, there is an insert titled: Antidepressant, noun (Concise Encyclopedia)—and delivers this definition to us:

(Please again read that on **The Menu as YOU EAT & Supporting References Pages**—on Pages 19 & 20)

MY SOLUTION

"Chinese herbology (simplified Chinese: 中药学; traditional Chinese: 中藥學; pinyin: zhōngyào xué) is the theory of traditional Chinese herbal therapy, which accounts for the majority of treatments in traditional Chinese medicine (TCM). The term herbology is misleading in so far as plant elements are by far the most commonly, but not solely used substances; animal, human, and mineral products are also utilized. Thus, the term "medicinal" (instead of herb) is usually preferred as a translation for 药 (pinyin: yào). Regarding Traditional Chinese herbal therapy, only few trials exist that are considered to be of adequate methodology by modern western medical researchers, and its effectiveness therefore is considered poorly documented.

"For example, a 2007 Cochrane review found promising evidence for the use of Chinese herbal medicine in relieving painful menstruation, compared to conventional medicine such as NSAIDs and the oral contraceptive pill, but the findings have to be interpreted with caution due to the generally low methodological quality of the included studies (as, amongst others, data for placebo control could not be obtained)." {http://en.wikipedia.org/wiki/Chinese_herbology}

Between my first consultation at a Herbal Medicine Clinic—on Friday, 26/10/12—to my most recent—Friday, 28/12/12—my crippling **Fatigue** symptoms have ineffably become like unuseable, **thermoelectric Energy** symptoms!!!!

MY CONCLUSION

OUR SUBJECTIVE HUMIDTEMP ENVIRONMENT

The inserted **HUMIDTEMP ENVIRONMENT** Charting below edits **MY** body's sensory response (in the third column) to the two **HUMIDTEMP FACTORS**—and their multiplicands—in the second column.

Another person [Person A], whom lives closer to the poles (and had adapted to a colder environment) might still feel the need to lower the temperature of his/her environment—and/or remove more clothing. Thus **Local HumidTemp Environment** will effectuate Person A's response:

Yet another person [Person Z], whom lives closer to the equator (and had adapted to a hotter environment) might still feel the need to raise the temperature of his/her environment—and/or don more clothing. Thus **Local HumidTemp Environment** will effectuate Person Z's response.

Humans can accommodate BOTH instances—that of a cold environment: and that of a hot environment—and still easily avoid illness and bizarre, monolithically grotesque side-effects!!

And hence **MY PERSONAL HUMIDTEMP ENVIRONMENTAL COUNTERPOISE** is also what is depicted directly below; where two earthy, natural, normal and physically-effecting, circumferent encompassing independent variables adjudicate our acceptation or renunciation—and subsequent espousal of or opposition to the environses of our geographic area.

HUMIDTEMP TEST #	ASSIGNING EACH OF THE TWO HUMIDTEMP FACTORS TO THEIR MULTIPLICANDS	DEFINING MY PERCEPTIVENESS OF THESE FOUR HUMIDTEMP ENVIRONMENTS ACCOUNTED FROM THEIR MULTIPLICATIVES
1	25°C x 45% = 1,125	BIT CHILLY
2	25°C x 46% = 1,150	NICE
3	26°C x 45% = 1,170	NICE
4	27°C x 46% = 1,242	NICE

OUR DEMANDED
MORALETHIC ENVIRONMENT

The below inserted **MORALETHIC ENVIRONMENT** Charting edits **OUR ONLY** acceptable sensory response (in the third column) to the two **MORALETHIC FACTORS**—and their multiplicands—in the second column.

All persons upon this earth [Persons A through to Persons Z], under the International Law of Human Rights, **MUST have FULL ACCESS** to these two **MORALETHIC FACTORS**.

Humans have the right to permit and should warrant and all humans should utterly conform to **ONLY** this unique and single instance.

And thus **OUR APPROVED MORALETHIC ENVIRONMENTAL COUNTERPOISE** is also what is depicted directly below:

MORALETHIC TEST #	ASSIGNING EACH OF THE TWO MORALETHIC FACTORS TO THEIR MULTIPLICANDS	DEFINING OUR PERCEPTIVENESS OF THE MORALETHIC ENVIRONMENT RESULTING FROM THE MULTIPLICATIVES
1 of 1	10/10 MORAL x 10/10 ETHIC = 100%	SATISFACTORY

Many human faces, from those of our precious, assailable, blameless kids' to our also-precious, conquerable, dignity-seeking grandparents'—mirror the dreadfully helpless plea for someone to understand their supplication—and rescue them from their current further-disadvantaged plight.

My thoughts are irresistibly, and emotively, double helixes towards each of those ones.

The World Is My Concern!!!

Bartholomew Identity.